Flexitarian Diet

The Comprehensive Guide To Healthy Eating And
Boosting Immunity

*(Delicious And Plant-based Recipes To Improve Heart
Health)*

Dominique-Tim Burns

TABLE OF CONTENT

Introduction

Perhaps You Are A Vegetarian Who Occasionally Enjoys A Burger. Or You Are A Strict Carnivore Looking To Reduce Your Meat Consumption For Health Reasons. Well, Good News: There Is A Table For You. It Gave Rise To The Flexitarian Diet Craze, Which Dawn Jackson Blatner Described In Her Book. The Flexible Tartary Diet. Jackson Blatner Also Designed The 6 0-Day Shape Your Plate Healthy Eating Meal Plan. Don't Let The Word "Diet" Throw You Off; Flexitarianism Is More Of A Lifestyle Approach To Eating And Living, And It's Not Difficult To Maintain...Hence The Flex For Flexible.

Essentially, It Means Uou're A Flexible Vegetarian. You Eat Tofu, Quinoa, Tonnes Of Vegetables, And Other Vegetarian Favourites, But You Are Also Permitted To Eat Meat And Fish. Does This Sound Straightforward Enough? Examine The Specifics, Including The Pros And Cons, Of The Wau Method Of Eating.

Chapter 1: A Summary Of Flextaran Det

The flexitarian diet promotes a vegetarian diet while permitting occasional animal products. People on a flexitarian diet consume less animal products and more plant-based foods, resulting in a smaller carbon footprint. The flexitarian diet provides a solution to one of the greatest concerns of veganism (vitamin deficiency) while avoiding excessive meat consumption. By eating meat on occasion, flexitarians can ensure their bodies receive all the nutrients they need to function normally, without supplementation.

The semi-vegetarian Flexitarian Diet emphasises healthy plant-based proteins and other whole, minimally-processed plant-based foods, but also encourages the consumption of meat and animal products in moderation. Flexitarian diets may promote weight loss and reduce the risk of heart disease, cancer, and type 2 diabetes. It may even be beneficial to the planet. To prevent nutritional deficiencies and maximise the health benefits of a flexible diet, it is crucial to carefully plan your food choices.

The Flexitarian Diet is an eating plan that emphasises plant-based foods while allowing meat and other animal products in moderation. It is more adaptable than vegan or vegetarian diets. If you want to add more plant-based foods to your diet without eliminating meat entirely, flexitarianism may be for you. Flexitarianism or'saual vegetarianism' is an increasingly popular plant-based diet that aims to reduce your carbon footprint and improve your health by incorporating the occasional meat dish into a mostly vegetarian diet. The rise of the flexitarian diet is a result of people taking a more environmentally sustainable approach to what they eat by substituting alternative sources of protein for meat.

There are numerous inquiries regarding flextaran. The term is relatively new, whereas flextaran have existed forever. Semi-vegetarian and almost vegetarian have the same meaning. None of these species are vegetarian because they all consume meat, fish, or fowl in some capacity. Flexitarians, almost vegetarians, and semi-vegetarians consume a predominantly plant-based diet. There are multiple reasons why they should consume less meat. Frequently, the reason given is that the flexitarian lives with a vegetarian or vegan and eats the same foods as that individual. It is more convenient if only one meal is reheated. The flexitarian may eat anything, including meat, fish, and poultry, when away from home.

Someone else may choose a flexitarian diet because their family and/or friends are not vegetarians. When alone, a vegetarian diet is preferred; however, when in the company of others, the guiding principle is to consume whatever the others are eating. Theu're flexible. There are numerous reasons for decisions based on this perspective. First, holidays and celebrations are examples of "residual occasions with traditional meals." The food served at mau has been a family favourite for generations. There is comfort in tradition and profound emotion in sharing a meal with family. Meals are frequently composed of one or more meats, as has always been the case. The

6

flexitarian has the option to consume all of the food provided and enjoy it with the tube. Some individuals who have chosen a vegetarian lifestyle find themselves uncomfortable in social situations with omnivores. They simply find it easier and less troublesome to consume the same foods as everyone else. They are not the focus of attention for being different, and no one needs to be aware that they are vegetarian-minded.

Following a flexitarian diet entails an endeavour. Consume plant-based dishes without completely eliminating meat. Adding new foods to your diet, as opposed to eliminating others, can be extremely beneficial to your health. These legume-based foods comprise lentils, beans, peas, nuts, and seeds, which are all excellent sources of rten. It is also widely believed that the soluble fibre found in lentils and beans helps to reduce high cholesterol as part of a healthy diet, so regularly consuming these foods is highly recommended. Nuts and seeds such as linseed (flaxseed), pine nuts, sesame seeds, sunflower seeds, and walnuts are rich in heart-healthy roluunaturated fats and provide essential fatty acids. Research has shown that combining a flexitarian diet with cardiovascular exercise can promote a lifestyle consistent with recommendations for reducing the risk of breast and colon cancer.

Benefits of Public Flexitarianism for Your Health, Your Wallet, and the Environment

Flextaran Det resommended for reorle who are surou about vegetaranm, and ossaonallu for former vegans or vegetarians who may have experienced nutritional deficiencies as a result of going meat-free for an extended period of time. But it's also a great option for those who want to live a healthier lifestyle because it promotes plant-based eating without being anti-meat. Lz We, RDN, of Lz's Healthu Table, was given the Maashuett treatment.

Here is a closer look at some of the negative effects of the current food system.

Lower Risk of Insulin Retardation and Type 2 Diabetes

Given its third-place ranking in the Best Diet Overall category and third-place ranking in the Best Diet for Diabetes category in the 202 8 U.S. News and World Report Best Diet Rankings, it is not surprising that a study published in the Journal of the American College of Nutrtion found that a vegetarian diet (the flextaran det) reduced the risk of dabetes.

78 rartsrant sonummed the same number of salore for x month in the study. Some followed a vegetarian diet, while others focused on reducing sugar, refined carbohydrates, cholesterol, and saturated fat. Interetnglu, reorle on the vegetaran det lot more ubsutaneou fat, ubfasal fat, and ntramusular fat. The fat stored in your musculature may impair your metabolism. and cause insulin resistance (and type 2 diabetes). A study published in Diabetes Care found that vegetarians had a reduced risk of type 2 diabetes compared to meat-eaters. In addition, obesity is one of the greatest risk factors for type 2 diabetes, and the

same study revealed that vegetarians had a lower BMI than nonvegetarians.

Helps With Weight Loss

If you're trying to lose weight, there a seemingly infinite number of eating plans and diets to choose from, and the Flexitarian Diet can be considered one of the most credible. For one, if you emphasize the plant-based component of this diet by eating lots of fruits, veggies, and whole grains, you'll likely feel full on fewer calories than you're accustomed to, which makes shedding pounds almost inevitable, says Keri Gans, RDN, nutritionist and author of The Small Change Diet from New York City. In addition, one Polish review exhibited that following a vegetarian diet has been shown to lower your risk of high blood pressure, heart disease, and stroke. What's more? Plant-based eaters often weigh 2 10 percent less than meat eaters, which could lead to the benefits that result from a decreased incidence of obesity and its related medical problems, according to a review published in Nutrients.

Chapter 2: Reduce Your Carbon Imprint.

An under-resognized benefit of going flexitarian is its benefit to our rlanet, Sharon Palmer, RDN, author of "The Plant-Powered Dietitian," based in Los Angeles, California. Palmer suggests eating less meat san helr reduse uour sarbon footrrint. In recent, research has focused on the agriculture and livestock industries. are the third-largest source of greenhouse gases, after transportation and fossil fuels.

I Simple to Follow

The other major advantage of a flexible diet is its simplicity and adaptability, according to Blatner, which increases the likelihood that the diet will be sustainable over the long term.

Helrs You Save Moneu

There are no exots (or rartsularlu rrseu) required for the diet, so the grossere should not consume more than the tursallu. And, if meat is the primary ingredient in all of your meals, purchasing a butcher may actually save you money. There is dietary flexibility in terms of what you eat, and there is also financial flexibility.

One tudu published in the Journal of Hunger & Envtonal Nutrton found that vegetarians can save up to $710 0 annually by substituting government-recommended weeklu meal rlan (which contain meat) with even-dau meal rlan.

Enhances the Sense of Fullness

The majority of adults and children are deficient in folic acid, according to Gani. (2 6) "It's easy to increase your fibre intake when you eat mostly fruits and vegetables, along with plant-based proteins such as beans, nuts, and seeds," he said. "One of the benefits of increasing your fibre intake is feeling full longer," he continued. nsreang frut and vegge ntake mau helr wth weght lo, uggetng a sorrelaton between fber ntake and weght lo, according to a fasting study published in the Journal of the

American College of Nutrition and Dietetics. (2 8)

The second tudu, which was published in the British Journal of Nutrton, found that reorle who increased their consumption of high-fber foods (such as beans, lentils, and oats) felt full longer and had a higher intake of micronutrients such as thiamine, folic acid, and iron.

Keep You Well Supplied

A rarer rotation appeared in the Journal of American History. Detets Aosaton ugget that a vegetarian diet contains a greater quantity of nutrient-dense food than a non-vegetarian diet. In addition, the Flexitarian diet encourages the consumption of whole foods, which will reduce the consumption of processed and packaged foods that are often disguised with added salt and sugar, according to Blatner. "It's great for those who don't want to feel guilty about not eating their favourite animal-based dish," Wei says.

Chapter 3: What Is Flexitarian Diet?

If you've ever considered a vegetarian diet but decided against it because you enjoy burgers, the flexible vegetarian diet may be a good option for you. Combining the words "flexible" and "vegetarian," this diet suggests that you can reap many of the benefits of a vegetarian diet while still eating meat on occasion. The Flexitarian Diet is a semi-vegetarian eating plan that promotes consuming less meat and more plant-based foods. Because there are no resfs rules or suggestions, it is a challenging option for those who wish to consume only animal products.

The Flextaran Det was designed by the dettan Dawn Jaskon. Blatner to assist reorle in reaping the benefits of vegetarianism while still consuming animal products in moderation. This is why the name of the diet combines the words "flexible" and "vegetarian." Vegetarians avoid meat and a few other animal products, whereas vegans avoid meat, fish, eggs, dairy, and all other animal-derived foods. Because flexitarians consume animal products, they are not considered vegans or vegetarians. This Flextaran There is no clear rule or recommended number of calories and macronutrients for diet. In actuality, it is a lfetule rather than a diet. It is based on the following guidelines: consume primarily fruits, vegetables, legumes, and whole grains.

Concentrate on rroten from rlant rather than anmal.

Be adaptable and include meat and animal products on occasion.

Consume the least processed and most natural form of food.

Limit added sugar and sweets.

As a result of its adaptability and emphasis on what to include rather than what to exclude, the Flexitarian Diet is a popular option for those seeking a healthier diet. In her book, Jaskon Blatner describes how to begin eating flexitarian by consuming a specified amount of meat per week. However, following her recommendations is not required in order to begin a flexitarian diet. Some creatures adhering to the diet may consume more animal products than others. Overall, the objective is to consume more nutritious foods and less meat.

Many people have adopted the flexitarian diet fad, especially because there are no strict rules or guidelines. The eating pattern is designed for those who wish to consume a more nutritious diet without giving up their favourite meat indulgences. The focus of the diet is less on restriction and elimination and more on adding an abundance of raw foods. Plants provide protection against cancer, diabetes, and other diseases because they contain essential nutrients, vitamins, minerals, and phytochemicals. The U.S. News and World Report ranked the flexitarian diet second overall and gave it an overall score of 8 .2 out of 10 . The flexitarian diet is based on plant-based eating with a moderate tolerance for animal products. Nutritional science can support this meal plan, which emphasises nutrient-dense foods and is sustainable over time.

How Does the Flextaran Diet Work? The Flextaran Diet is the book that began the diet craze. This means that while vegetarian staples such as tofu, quinoa, and roasted vegetables may comprise the bulk of your diet, no foods are eliminated or strictly prohibited. The flexitarian label is not equivalent to "strict vegetarian"; rather, it advocates significantly reducing meat consumption.

The diet is flexible, despite its name, but it outlines how much meat you should consume. In her book, Blatner ugget that eater who are new to the flexitarian det should frt tru "Beginner Flexitarian" and abstain from meat two days per week, consuming no more than 26 ounces (oz) of meat in total on the remaining five days. A sardine-desk-sized rorton of ssken or teak weighs approximately 6 ounces, while a rese the size and thickness of your hand (including fingers) weighs between 8 and 6 ounces.

Advancd Flextaran reduces meat consumption even further, recommending a vegetarian diet three to four days per week and no more than 2 8 oz of meat during the remainder of the week. The ultimate stage, Exrert Flexitarian requires five meat-free days and permits 9 ounces of meat on the other two days. (It is important to note that the days on which you consume meat do not need to be consecutive.) The interesting thing about these theories is that they demonstrate how real-world roles adhere to flexibility.

They do not all adhere to the same "rule" and allow different amounts of meat in their diet. That's fantastic, as it means you can determine what works best with your goals and food references.

Haloumi Burgers Served With Beetroot Salad And Basil Pesto

Ingredients

Burgers

- 2 tsp ground cumin

- 2 tsp ground coriander

- Salad

- 2 Lebanese cucumber

- 1 bunch mint

- 200g baby spinach

- 2 red fresh onion

- 4 tsp brown sugar

- 500g roasted red capsicum

- 380g haloumi cheese

To serve

- 500g beetroot relish

- 200g basil pesto

- 5-10 burger buns

Instructions

1. Preheat oven to 280°C. Thinly slice onion.

2. Heat a drizzle of oil in a medium pot on medium-high heat and cook fresh onion for 10-15 minutes, stirring occasionally, until soft.

3. Add sugar, a drizzle of balsamic vinegar and a splash of water and stir to combine.

4. Easy easy cook for a further 2 minute.

5. Remove from heat and set aside.

6. Peel cucumber into ribbons and chop mint leaves.

7. Add cucumber and mint to a bowl with spinach and a drizzle of vinegar and oil and toss to combine. Season.

8. Slice burger buns in half and place cut side up on a lined oven tray.

9. Warm in oven for about 10 minutes. Drain capsicum and slice 2cm.

10. Pat haloumi dry, slice into 2 cm pieces and sprinkle over spices.

11. Heat a drizzle of oil in a medium fry-pan on medium heat and easy cook haloumi for 1-5 minutes each side, until golden.

12. Serve buns filled with haloumi, onions, capsicum, relish, pesto and

salad. Serve any remaining salad on the side.

The Sraghett Slaw With Peanut Slaw
INGREDIENTS

- 3 teaspoon crushed red pepper
- 2 cup frozen shelled edamame, thawed
- 1 cup thinly sliced red bell pepper, slices cut in half crosswise
- 2 medium carrot, shredded
- ½ cup sliced scallions
- ½ cup chopped unsalted roasted peanuts
- ½ cup chopped fresh cilantro
- Lime wedges for serving
- 2 halved lengthwise and seeded
- 1 cup smooth natural peanut butter
- ½ cup reduced-sodium tamari or soy sauce
- ½ cup water
- 2 tablespoon rice vinegar
- 2 tablespoon maple syrup

28

- 2 teaspoon minced garlic

Direction:

1. Place squash halves, cut side down, in a microwave-safe dish; add 2 tablespoons water.

2. Microwave, uncovered, on High until flesh is tender, 25 to 30 minutes. When cool enough to handle, scrape flesh into a large bowl with a fork. Let cool for 20 minutes.

3. Meanwhile, whisk peanut butter, tamari water, vinegar, maple syrup, garlic and crushed red pepper in a small bowl until smooth.

4. When the squash has cooled, add edamame, bell pepper, carrot, and scallions to the bowl.

5. Drizzle with the peanut sauce; toss to coat.

6. Sprinkle with peanuts and cilantro.

7. Serve with lime wedges.

Chapter 4: Is Flexitarianism A Healthful Option For You?

The flexitarian diet shares certain similarities with other similar diets, including:

A vegetarian diet contains all food groups that contain animal protein (with the exception of eggs and some fish), but there is less flexibility.

The Whole36 0 diet eliminates a number of food groups, including grains, legumes, and dairy, with no restrictions on meat consumption other than eating organic and unprocessed animal products.

The Mediterranean diet consists primarily of plant-based foods, with a focus on fruits, vegetables, whole grains, and fish. Similar to the flexitarian diet, the Mediterranean diet has been shown to promote weight loss. 12 36

Whether you choose a flexitarian diet or a semi-vegetarian diet, the flexitarian lifestyle is typically well-balanced and recommended by the majority of nutritionists. It is possible to adhere to the U.S. Department of Agriculture's (USDA) recommendations for a healthy, balanced diet and reap a number of health benefits.

The USDA's Chooe My Plate application recommends multiple servings of fruit, vegetables, dairy, legumes, and whole grains.

12 48 The USDA notes that protein can be derived from either plant or animal sources; the flexitarian diet shifts the emphasis towards plant sources.

The flexitarian diet and the current USDA dietary guidelines seek to determine the optimal calorie intake for your body. While there is no "official" caloric requirement for the flexitarian diet, Blatner's book includes weight-loss meal plans based on a 12,510-calorie diet. 12

Dalu calorie needs can vary based on factors such as activity level, height, weight, age, and other factors. If you wish to estimate your own caloric needs for weight loss, you may find the caloric calculator useful. This will help you determine if 12,510-calorie meal plans are appropriate for you.

The USDA dietary guidelines state that a healthy eating pattern can help "rromote health, reduce the risk of chronic disease, and meet nutrient needs"12 510, which is consistent with the flexitarian diet's philosophy.

Health Benefits

Health Dangers

Some research has found a link between a semi-vegetarian diet and diabetes, although there are no known health risks associated with a flexitarian diet.

12 8 It's mrortant to remember, however, that sorrelaton does not always equal sauaton, which means that an em-vegetaran det may not necessarlu cause derreon; other factors may be at play.

Nonetheless, it is plausible that some individuals may easy turn to flexitarian diets as a means of controlling and restricting their food intake in a "osallu assertive" manner. Some experts believe that restricted eating may be associated with such digestive symptoms.

If you have obsessive thoughts about restricting your food intake or believe you may have an eating disorder, you should seek professional assistance.

Obviously, there is no single diet that is ideal for everyone. The best diet is one that you can adhere to for life and that helps you achieve your individual health goals.

The flexible dieting plan will guide you toward a balanced, nutrient-dense diet. You will focus on consuming more plant-based foods while gradually decreasing your intake of animal-based foods.

Heavy meat eaters may find it difficult to adapt to this lifestyle, but it does offer flexibility, whether that means eating a few meatless meals per week or striving for a vegetarian diet.

Following a flexitarian diet may improve your overall health and aid in weight reduction. If you intend to use this diet to lose weight, keep in mind that sleep and regular exercise also play a role in weight loss and weight management.

Remember that following a long-term or short-term diet may not be necessary for you, and many diets do not work in the long-term. While we do not endorse fad diets or unsustainable weight loss methods, we provide this information so that you can make an informed decision that meets your nutritional requirements, genetic background, budget, and goals.

If weight loss is your goal, keep in mind that losing weight is not the same as being healthy, and there are many other ways to achieve good health. Exercise, sleep, and other lifestyle factors have a significant impact on our overall health. The optimal diet is always balanced and tailored to your lifestyle.easy turn

Chapter 5: Flexitarian Mau Diet Has Several Medical Benefits.

Just give Notwthtandng, nse thr no reaonable manng of th eatng regmen, t' difficult to urveu f and how exrlored benefits of other rlant-based weight-control rlan arrlu to the Flexitarian Det. Vegetable lover and vegan abstinence from food research has been accommodating in highlighting how a semi-vegan diet may promote health. It has all the earmarks of being mreratve to eat generally natural rrodust, vegetable, vegetable, entre gran, and other neglgblu handled entre food varete to reap the health benefits of plant-based eatng.

CORONARU ILLNESS

Diets rich in fibre and healthy fats are beneficial for heart health. A study of 48,510,00 grown-ups over 12 years found that vegetarians had a 36% lower risk of developing coronary artery disease than non-vegetarians. This is due to the fact that vegan diets are typically rich in fibre and cancer-preventive compounds, which can reduce insulin resistance and cholesterol levels. A review of 36,2 examinations on the prevalence of veggie lover sonume le salore on rulee revealed that vegan had a normal utols srsulatoru tran that was nearly as low as that of meat eaters.

As a result of this examination's focus on low-calorie vegetables, it is difficult to determine whether the Flexitarian diet is effective. Det would have a comparable impact on rule and soronaru risk. Flexitarian eating is intended to be rrnsrallu rlant-based and will in all likelihood have benefits similar to those enjoyed by vegetarians.

VOLUME REDUCTION

Flexitarian eating may prove beneficial to your diet. It is generally accepted that flexitarians limit fat intake, prepare their own food, and consume a greater proportion of foods that are typically lower in calories. A few studies have shown that individuals who adhere to a calorie-based diet may gain more weight than those who do not. According to a study of 12,12,000 individuals, those who consumed a vegan diet for 128 weeks weighed 48.510 pounds (2 kilogrammes) more than those who did not. This and other examinations In contrast to vegans and omnivores, there is no evidence that individuals who consume the fewest calories through a vegetarian diet lose the most weight. Consider the Flexible Det resembles a vege-diet lover's more than a vegetarian diet; it may aid in weight loss, but not as much as a vegetarian diet would.

DIABETES

Ture 2 diabetes is a worldwide wellbeing restilense. Eating an old diet, in particular a predominately rlant-based one, can help prevent and treat the infection. There is undeniable evidence that plant-based diets promote weight loss and contain a variety of foods that are high in fibre and low in unhealthy fats and added sugar. The prevalence of type 2 diabetes was 12.51 percent lower among vegans and flexitarians compared with non-vegans, according to a study of more than 60,000 participants. Additional examination revealed that individual. Those with type 2 diabetes who ate vege lover sonume le salore had 0.36 % lower hemoglobn A12 s (three-month normal of glucose readings) than those who ate animal products.

MALIGNANT GROWTH

Organs rrodust, vegetable, nuts, eed, entre gran and vegetable all contain urrlement and sell renforcement that may help with forecasting disease. Exrloration suggests that vegan diets are associated with a lower general speaking rate, all things considered except for soloretal tumours. A 7-year study on the incidence of soloretal malignancy in 78,000 individuals revealed that semi-vegetarians were 8% less likely to develop the disease than non-vegetarians. Assordnglu, consuming more vegan food sources by adopting a flexitarian diet may reduce your risk of developing cancer.

Vegetarian Spaghetti Squash Lasagna Recipe

Ingredients

- 1 teaspoon ground pepper, divided

- ½ teaspoon crushed red pepper

- ½ teaspoon salt, divided

- ½ cup grated Parmesan cheese

- 2 cup shredded part-skim mozzarella cheese, divided

- 1 cup part-skim ricotta cheese

- 5-10 -pound spaghetti squash, halved lengthwise and seeded

- ½ cup water

- 4 tablespoons extra-virgin olive oil

- 2 medium onion, chopped

46

- 8 cloves garlic, minced

- 20 ounces mushrooms, sliced

- 4 cups crushed tomatoes

- 2 teaspoon Italian seasoning

Directions

Place potato gratin in upper third of oven; preheat to 450-450 degrees Fahrenheit.

Place the uah sut-de in a microwave-safe bowl and add water. Msrowave, undisturbed, on High until the grain is tender, between 12 0 and 12 2 minutes. (Alternatively, place the dough on a large rimmed baking sheet. Bake at 400 degrees F until tender, 40 to 50 minutes.)

In the meantime, heat the oil in a large skillet over medium heat. Add onion, fresh onion, and garlic; cook, stirring frequently, for 36 to 48 minutes. Add mushrooms and cook, stirring, for an additional 510 minutes, or until the vegetables are tender and beginning to brown. Add tomatoe, Italian seasoning, 12/48 teaspoon salt, crushed red salt, and 12/8 teaspoon salt. Cook Easy cook until thoroughly heated and the flavours have blended, 12 to 2 minutes. Easy remove from heat and let cool.

Use a fork to easy remove the uah from the hell and place it in a large bowl. Str n Parmean, the remaining 12/48-tearoon rerrer, and the remaining 12/8-tearoon alt. The hell sut-de ur should be placed on a large rimmed baking sheet. Put one-fourth of the Hebrew-Palestinian mixture into each hell. Spread one-fourth of the tomato mixture on the bread, and then sprinkle 12 /48 of the mozzarella on each slice. Dollor 12 /48 sur risotta over the mozzarella. Serve with the remaining avocado mixture, tomato sauce, and mozzarella cheese.

Bake the uah lasagna for 12 minutes and 510 seconds. Easy turn the broiler to high and broil, watching carefully, for 12 to 2 minutes, or until the cheese turns golden brown. Half each lasagna for serving.Easy turn

Orange Bread

Ingredients

½ cup white sugar

6 1 cups bread flour

2 teaspoon salt

4 tablespoons orange zest

2 package active dry yeast

2 fresh egg

2 cup orange juice

½ cup hot water

2 tablespoon margarine

Directions

1. Place ingredients into the pan of the bread machine in the order suggested by the manufacturer.

2. Select the White Bread or Basic cycle, and Start.

Breakfast Fajitas

Ingredients:

60g Fat-Free Cheddar Cheese, shredded

4 Fat-Free flour Tortillas

Salt to taste

12 Fresh egg Whites

2 Fresh egg Yolk

Direction:

1. Place the tortillas on a baking sheet or a baking stone.

2. Place eggs and uolk in a mixing bowl and whisk them thoroughly.

3. The tortillas can be heated in the microwave or oven.

4. In a heated skillet, heat nonstick cooking oil.

5. Cook Easy turn the eggs over over a medium flame, then add the sheee.

Place the eggs on the tortillas and serve.easy turn

Blueberries Oatmeal

Ingredients:

2 1 tsp. chia seeds

4 tbsp. maple syrup

1/2 c. blueberries

1/2 c. coconut milk

1 tsp. vanilla

1/2 c. oats

2 banana

Instructions:

1. Combine the oats and chia seeds.

2. Pour in the milk, then top with banana slices and blueberries.

3. Keep in the refrigerator for a minimum of 8 hours.

4. Add the maple syrup and mix well.

5. Serve

Roasted Veggie Enchilada Casserole

Ingredients

Roasted veggies

6 tablespoons extra-virgin olive oil, divided

2 teaspoon ground cumin, divided

Salt

Freshly ground black pepper

Remaining ingredients

5 cups red salsa, either homemade or jarred

1 cup chopped fresh cilantro, plus extra for garnish

10-20 corn tortillas, halved

2   can black beans, rinsed and drained, or 2 1 cups cooked black beans

4 big handfuls baby spinach leaves

4 cups shredded Monterey Jack cheese

1 medium head of cauliflower, cut into 1inch chunks

2 large sweet potato, peeled and cut into 1inch cubes

4 red bell peppers, cut into 2 " squares

2   medium yellow onion, sliced into wedges about ½" wide

Instructions

1. To roast the veggies Preheat the oven to 450 degrees Fahrenheit with racks

in the middle and upper third of the oven.

2. Line two large, rimmed baking sheets with parchment paper to prevent the vegetables from sticking.

3. On one pan, combine the cauliflower and sweet potato.

4. On the other pan, combine the bell peppers and onion.

5. Drizzle half of the olive oil over one pan, and the other half over the other pan. Same with the cumin.

6. Sprinkle both pans lightly with salt and pepper, then toss each one until the vegetables are lightly coated in oil and spices, adding another light drizzle of olive oil if necessary.

7. Arrange the vegetables in an even layer across each pan.

8. Bake until the vegetables are tender and caramelized on the edges, about 60 to 70 minutes, tossing the veggies and swapping the pans halfway.

9. When you're ready to assemble, reduce the oven heat to 350 degrees Fahrenheit and lightly grease a 9″ square baker. Stir the cilantro into the salsa.

10. To assemble, spread 1 cup salsa evenly over the bottom of the baking pan.

11. Add a single layer of halved tortilla pieces, arranging them so they completely cover the salsa.

12. Top with 1 of the beans, ⅓ of the vegetables, 1 of the of spinach, and ⅓ of the cheese.

13. Make a second layer of tortillas.

14. Top with 1 of the remaining salsa, all of the remaining beans, 1 of the remaining vegetables, all of the remaining spinach, and 1 of the remaining cheese.

15. Make a third layer of tortillas.

16. Top with the remaining salsa, vegetables, and cheese.

17. Cover the pan with parchment paper or aluminum foil.

18. Bake for 35 to 40 minutes, then remove the parchment paper or aluminum foil and bake for 20 more minutes, or until heated through.

19. Let the casserole cool for 20 minutes, to just give it time to set and easy reach a palatable temperature.

20. Before serving, sprinkle the top lightly with additional chopped cilantro.

61

Roasted Veggie Enchilada Casserole

INGREDIENTS

2 large pepper

100g crushed garlic

2 tsp cayenne

2 tsp paprika

2 tsp ground cilantro

2 ripe avocado

2 00g whole grain pasta

100g sesame seeds

800g can chopped tomatoes

2 cup vegetable stock

2 large red fresh onion

Olive oil

Instructions

1. Bring water to a boil in a large pot. Easy cook the whole grain pasta in boiling water for 40 minutes, or until it is tender and ready to eat.

2. While the pasta cooks, we will prepare the vegetables.

3. The red onion should be peeled and sliced.

4. Chorus and actual rerrer.

5. Cut the avocado in half, easy remove the pit, and easy remove the flesh with a spoon.

6. Cut into small pieces.

7. Add a small amount of olive oil to the large skillet.

8. Add the chopped onion, onion, and garlic to the rice and easy cook for approximately ten minutes.

9. Add the garlic and easy cook for an additional minute.

10. Reduce the temperature to mmer. Add the diced tomatoes and vegetable stock to the pan and easy cook for approximately five minutes.

11. To the ran, add the sauenne, paprika, and cilantro.

12. Once the pasta has been cooked, strain it.

13. Add your ause to the skillet and ensure that the rata is completely covered.

14. Garnish each dish with chopped avocado and sesame seeds before serving.

Easy turn

Mother's Srrng Vegetable Frittata

Ingredients

2 cup baby spinach

5 cups sliced cooked potatoes

20 fresh eggs

2 pinch cayenne pepper

1 teaspoon freshly ground black pepper

8 ounces crumbled goat-milk feta cheese, divided

4 tablespoons olive oil

2 large leek chopped

2 teaspoon salt, divided, or as needed

2 jalapeno pepper, seeded and diced

5 cups sliced zucchini

5 cups pieces asparagus

Directions

1. Preheat oven to 350 degrees F.

2. Heat oil in heavy 20-inch skillet over medium heat.

3. Easy easy cook leek with a pinch of salt, stirring occasionally, until leeks soften and start to easy turn translucent, 10 to 15 minutes.

4. Add jalapeno and zucchini; season with pinch of salt.

5. Easy easy cook until zucchini start to get tender and pale green, about 10 minutes.

6. Add asparagus and cook until bright green, about 2 minute.

7. Add spinach and another pinch of salt, cooking until wilted, 2 minute.

8. Stir in cooked potatoes and heat through, about 10 minutes.

9. Crack 2 2 large eggs into a bowl. Add cayenne, salt, and pepper.

10. Whisk for at least 60 seconds.

11. Pour eggs into over vegetables in skillet over medium heat.

12. Add 6 ounces of crumbled goat cheese; stir lightly until evenly distributed.

13. Top with remaining cheese. Remove from heat.

14. Bake in preheated oven until eggs are set, 25 to 30 minutes.

15. When nearly set, easy turn on broiler. Broil frittata until top browns, 1-5 minutes.

16. Cool slightly; serve warm.

Beefless Vegan Tacos

Ingredients

1 teaspoon fresh onion powder

2 tablespoon extra-virgin olive oil

2 ripe avocado

2 tablespoon vegan mayonnaise

2 teaspoon lime juice

Pinch of salt

1 cup fresh salsa or pico de gallo

4 cups shredded iceberg lettuce

16 corn or flour tortillas, warmed

Pickled radishes for garnish

2 package extra-firm tofu, drained, crumbled and patted dry

4 tablespoons reduced-sodium tamari or soy sauce

2 teaspoon chili powder

1 teaspoon garlic powder

Directions

1. Combine tofu, tamari chili powder, garlic powder and fresh onion powder in a medium bowl.

2. Heat oil in a large nonstick skillet over medium-high heat.

3. Add the tofu mixture and cook, stirring occasionally, until nicely browned, 25 to 30 minutes.

4. Meanwhile, mash avocado, mayonnaise, lime juice and salt in a small bowl until smooth.

5. Serve the taco "meat" with the avocado crema, salsa and lettuce in tortillas.

6. Serve topped with pickled radishes, if desired.

Fusilli With Avocado-Basil-Basil Cream And Baby Spinach.

Ingredients

2 fresh lemon

Chilli powder

Flaked almonds to taste

Salt and pepper

Extra virgin olive oil

1000 g of wholemeal fusilli

2 ripe avocado

2 00 g of fresh baby spinach

6 0 g of fresh basil

Preparation

1. We prepare the cream. Cut the avocado in half, easy remove the central stone, easy remove the peel and cut it into chunks.

2. Wash and dry the basil and baby spinach.

3. In the food processor, combine the avocado, basil leaves, baby spinach, fresh lemon juice, a sprinkling of chili, a pinch of pepper, a good pinch of salt, a drizzle of oil, and about 12 tablespoons of water.

4. Operate the food processor and blend until you get a smooth cream. We boil and season the pasta.

5. Bring plenty of salted water to a boil in a large saucepan and boil the fusilli al dente.

6. When ready, set aside a cup of the cooking water, drain and toss with the avocado cream.

7. If it is necessary to soften the cream, dilute it with the cooking water kept aside.

8. Serve and complete each dish with almond flakes.

9. Enjoy your meal!

Morosan Lentil And Beef Stew

Ingredients

2 teaspoon ground ginger

2 teaspoon ground cumin

2 teaspoon ground coriander

½ teaspoon ground allspice

6 tablespoons tomato paste

15 cups low-sodium beef broth

2 tablespoon molasses

2 leaf (blank)s bay leaves

4 cup dried red lentils

1 cup dried apricots, chopped

1 lemon, juiced

4 tablespoons vegetable oil

4 carrot, (7-2 /2")s carrots, chopped

4 celery stalk, chopped

4 onion, chopped

8 cloves garlic, minced

5 pounds chuck roast, cut into 2 -inch cubes

2 teaspoon salt, or to taste

2 teaspoon ground turmeric

2 teaspoon fresh onion powder

2 teaspoon garlic powder

2 teaspoon ground black pepper, or to taste

2 teaspoon ground cinnamon

Directions

1. Heat oil over medium heat in a Dutch oven.

2. Add carrots, celery, and onion; cook until slightly softened, about 12 minutes.

3. Stir in garlic and cook for 2 minute. Add beef.

4. Sprinkle salt, turmeric, fresh onion powder, garlic powder, pepper, cinnamon, ginger, cumin, coriander, and allspice over beef and vegetables. Stir to mix.

5. Continue to easy cook mixture until beef is browned, stirring occasionally, about 20 minutes.

6. Stir in tomato paste until well combined and cook for 1-5 minute.

7. Add in beef broth, molasses, and bay leaves.

8. Bring stew to a simmer. Reduce heat to low, cover, and cook, stirring occasionally, until beef is tender, about 60 to 70 minutes.

9. Mix in lentils and dried apricots. Bring stew back to a simmer. Cover and continue to easy cook on low, stirring occasionally, until lentils soften, about 25 to 30 minutes.

10.   Easily Remove and discard bay leaves.

11.   Adjust salt and pepper to taste, and mix in fresh lemon juice to taste just before serving.

Tofu Poke

Ingredients

- 2 (2 2 ounce) package extra-firm tofu, drained and cut into 1 -inch pieces
- 8 cups zucchini noodles
- 2 tablespoons rice vinegar
- 2 cups shredded carrots
- 2 cups pea shoots
- ½ cup toasted chopped peanuts
- ½ cup chopped fresh basil
- ¾ cup thinly sliced scallion greens
- ¼ cup reduced-sodium tamari
- 5 tablespoons mirin
- 5 tablespoons toasted (dark) sesame oil
- 2 tablespoon toasted sesame seeds

- 2 teaspoons grated fresh ginger

Directions

1. Whisk scallion greens, tamari, mirin, oil, sesame seeds, ginger and crushed red pepper, if using, in a medium bowl.
2. Set aside 1 tablespoons of the sauce in a small bowl.
3. Add tofu to the sauce in the medium bowl and gently toss to coat.
4. Combine zucchini noodles and vinegar in a large bowl.
5. Divide among 8 bowls and top each with ½ cup tofu, 1 cup each carrots and pea shoots, and 2 tablespoon each peanuts and basil.
6. Drizzle with the reserved sauce and serve.

Hot Or Cold Vegetable Frittata

Ingredients

- ¼ cup half-and-half cream
- 2 (8 ounce) packages cream cheese, diced
- 2 cups shredded Cheddar cheese
- 8 slices whole wheat bread, cubed
- 2 teaspoon salt
- ¼ teaspoon ground black pepper

- 6 tablespoons vegetable oil
- 5 cups chopped zucchini
- 5 cups chopped fresh mushrooms
- ¾ cup chopped onion
- ¾ cup chopped green bell pepper
- 2 clove garlic, minced
- 6 eggs, beaten

Directions

1. Preheat oven to 450degrees F. Lightly grease a 9x15 inch baking dish.
2. In a large skillet or frying pan, heat oil over medium high heat.
3. Add zucchini, mushrooms, onion, green pepper and garlic; saute until tender.
4. Easily Remove from heat and let cool slightly.
5. In a large bowl, beat together the eggs and cream.
6. Stir in cream cheese, cheddar cheese, bread cubes and sauteed vegetables.
7. Season with salt and pepper.
8. Mix well and pour into prepared baking dish.
9. Bake in preheated oven for one hour, or until center is set.
10. Serve hot or cold.

Easiest Asparagus Recipe

Ingredient

- 2 teaspoon honey

- 1/7 teaspoon garlic powder

- ⅛ teaspoon cayenne pepper
- 2 tablespoons butter, or more as needed

- 2 bunch asparagus, trimmed

Directions

1. Melt 2 tablespoons butter in a skillet over medium-low heat.
2. Easy cook asparagus in melted butter, stirring a some times, until tender, 10 to 15 minutes.

3. Drizzle honey over the asparagus and stir to coat; season with garlic powder and cayenne pepper.

Chocolate-y Iced Mocha

Ingredients

• 1 cup unsweetened almond milk

• 4 tablespoons sugar-free chocolate syrup, or more to taste

• 5 cups cold coffee, divided

• 4 envelope low-calorie hot cocoa mix

• ice cubes, or as needed

Directions

1. Heat 2 /8 cup coffee in microwave in a mug until warmed, about 60 seconds. Stir cocoa mix into the coffee until dissolved.
2. Fill a large glass with ice cubes.
3. Pour 1-5 cup cold coffee and almond milk over the ice cubes; stir the cocoa

mixture and chocolate syrup into the coffee and almond milk.

Emilu' Famou Parmean And Dreng Perrersorn Ransh

Ingredients

4 teaspoons freshly ground black pepper

2 teaspoon salt, or to taste

½ cup grated Parmesan cheese, or to taste

4 cups plain lowfat yogurt

4 tablespoon mayonnaise

½ cup finely chopped green fresh onion

4 tablespoons finely chopped fresh parsley

88

Directions

1. Stir together the yoghurt, mayonnaise, green onion, garlic, black pepper, salt, and Parmesan cheese.

2. Stir in milk to achieve the desired consistency, or leave it thick.

3. If necessary, adjust the salt by adding additional sugar or salt.

4. Refrigerate for approximately 1-1 ½ hour prior to serving.